Sleeping Disorders: How to Fall Asleep Quickly & Cure Insomnia

BY

PAUL STEPHENS

Table of Contents

Introduction

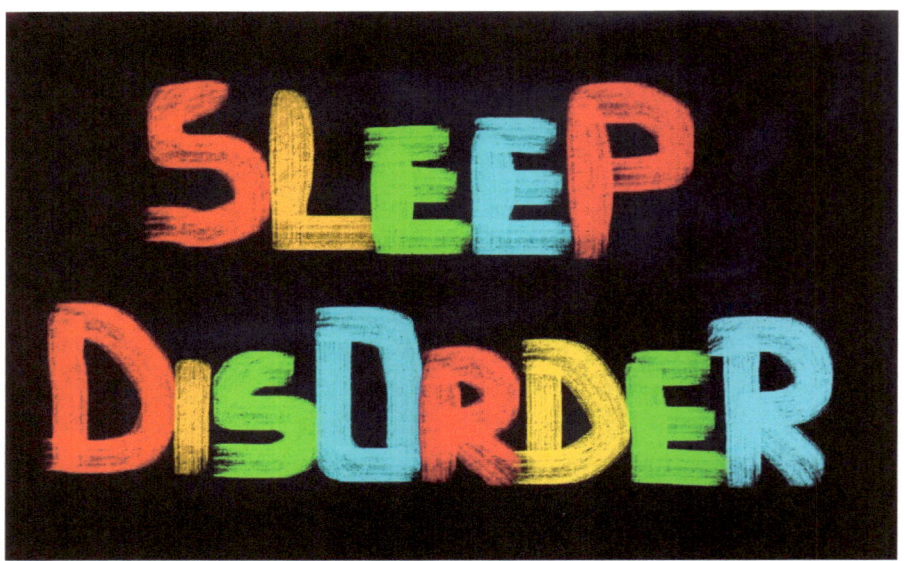

Insomnia

The inability to sleep is known as 'insomnia' and as many as half of us will suffer from it during our lifetimes, perhaps because we had a cup of coffee too many or something is stressing us out. Short-term kind of insomnia, known as 'acute insomnia' is a pain but shouldn't worry us too much. Yes, it's frustrating when you're going through it, but generally it goes away on its own; though taking some proactive steps like improving your sleep hygiene might help. It's the other kind of insomnia, what is known as 'chronic insomnia', which is the real joy killer. And we mean that quite literally, for sleep is a vital part for emotional balance and wellbeing.

It is towards this form of insomnia that this book is largely directed, because contrary to what you may have been led to believe, you can do something about it without needing to grab the pill bottle. Sleep is a far more involved and complex subject than you may have been led to believe. We still don't know all the ins and outs about it – for example, we don't actually know why we do it! But we are starting to get a pretty decent idea of how we can promote it and how you can hinder it.

Moreover, sleep is simply too important for you not to do something to improve yours. This is even true for people who don't regularly suffer from insomnia. The truth is quite a few of us could do with better quality sleep (to not even mention more of it!).

How to use this book?

This book will start out by exploring what both sleep and insomnia are, which might be a little bit theoretical for some, but will give you a better understanding of the how and why, which in turn might well be beneficial for fighting off the insomnia demons. This section also includes how much sleep we should get, what might be causing our insomnia and what happens to us as a result of sleep deprivation.

From there we will explore something known as a sleep diary. It isn't a very long section, but its value far outweighs its length, for through it you'll get a much better understanding of what is and isn't making you sleep poorly. Don't skip over this section! Instead, print it out and fill it out. It isn't a lot of work (it has, in fact, been designed to not take more than five minutes in the evening and the morning) and the benefits could be tremendous.

After that we'll be tackling actual sleep hygiene. This is where we'll discuss what you should change in your day to day life to improve the quality of your sleep. It can also be described as a list of 'dos and don'ts' and after that we'll slowly be looking at something called sleep apnea, which isn't insomnia but can negatively affect your sleep all the same.

Is this book only for insomniacs?

No it is not. Instead, it is for anybody who would like to improve the quality of their sleep. The sleep hygiene section, for example, can be beneficial to anybody. At the same time, this book is mainly geared towards those with insomnia and as such not all the sections will be equally useful to people who don't actually suffer from this dread disease (no it often isn't actually a disease, we just like the sound of 'dread disease', that's all).

Those people just looking to improve the quality of their sleep should instead focus their attention on the second half of the book – from the sleep diary onwards, really. In truth, nearly anybody can benefit from the sleep hygiene section as we all no doubt commit some of these sleep deprivation sins.

Chapter 1: What Is Sleep?

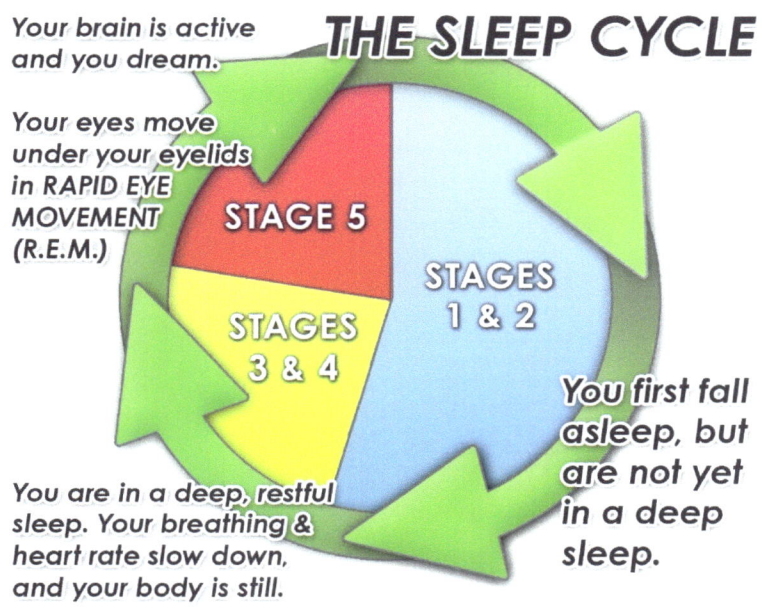

THE SLEEP CYCLE

Your brain is active and you dream.

Your eyes move under your eyelids in RAPID EYE MOVEMENT (R.E.M.)

STAGE 5

STAGES 3 & 4

STAGES 1 & 2

You first fall asleep, but are not yet in a deep sleep.

You are in a deep, restful sleep. Your breathing & heart rate slow down, and your body is still.

Even some of the more basic animals, like fruit flies and microscopic nematode worms sleep[1]. It's something built into all mammals, certainly, and many other animals as well, including birds. Dinosaurs might even have done it and it seems to be essential for our wellbeing. Why else would we have evolved to do it? After all, the disadvantage of having to shut your eyes and stop being alert to your surroundings for a good chunk of every day has significant drawbacks when there are predators on lurking. What it certainly is not for is conserving energy or because we have nothing better to do. The costs of being caught unaware are just too significant for that.

---

[1] http://www.bbc.com/earth/story/20160317-what-is-the-real-reason-we-sleep

The problem is that sleep has too many benefits for us to really know. For example, it helps memory storage, skill learning, mental recuperation and wellbeing, emotional regulation, our sex lives, physical recuperation and more. But just because it is good for that doesn't mean it is for that. After all, fingers are fantastic for picking your nose, but few people would argue that's why evolution gave them to us. And that's part of the reason there is no academic consensus – which is actually quite an incredible thing to say in this age of ubiquitous global communication and robots on mars. And yet it's true.

Stages of Sleep

Of course this doesn't mean we don't understand anything about sleep. For example, we understand there are five stages (or four) that we cycle through every single night. These are referred to, excitingly enough, as stage 1 through stage 5 (or 4). Scientists really do have a gift for naming things, don't they?

Stage 1. This is a light stage of sleep where your muscles relax and though your consciousness has winked out, it hasn't been completely turned off. Your eyes still move about (not to be mistaken by Rapid Eye Movement, which comes later) and your muscles might twitch. It is quite easy to wake you during this stage of sleep. This is also where you're likely to experience that falling sensation that has you suddenly jerk awake. This is because your muscles are relaxing which – if it happens too fast – can be interpreted by the body as meaning that you're dying. Your body then jerks you back to consciousness – a bit like those paddles in TV series use to make your heart restart. Don't worry, you're not actually dying. Our brains are just being overly careful, that's all.

Stage 2. Now you're entering proper sleep territory. Your eyes stop moving and your brain waves slow right down, though you can still experience bursts of brain activity.

Stage 3. Here your brain waves are mainly something called 'Delta waves', interspersed with occasionally shorter, more active waves. This is the first stage that is referred to as 'deep sleep'.

Stage 4. This stage continues your deep sleep – or delta – sleep stage. Here your body and brain are the closest to turn off for the night, though in no way is your brain shut down. Both stage 3 and stage 4 are difficult stages to wake somebody up from. Recently scientists in the US did away with the difference between stage 3 and 4 entirely, fusing them together into one overarching stage. No, these are not the same scientists that got rid of the planet Pluto.

Stage 5. Also known as the REM or rapid eye movement stage, this is where most of your dreaming occurs. At this point your muscles become paralyzed (so that you don't thrash about wildly and hit people) and your eyes twitch from side to side. In some ways you are probably the closest you've been to being awake since stage 1 here, with brain waves actually matching your waking state, breathing being shallow and your heart rate increasing. In the past this was known as 'paradoxical sleep' as there was very little to differentiate this stage from your waking stage in a brain scanner. We now know that is because it is here that you are processing a lot of the material that you picked up throughout the day for permanent storage. Interestingly enough, this is the most recently evolved state. "If there's a new kid on the block it's REM sleep," says Matthew Walker from Berkley University.

Normally, you cycle through these five (or four) stages once or twice per night. During this time, you'll only spend about an hour and a half to two hours in the REM stage of sleep. Yes, it feels like a lot more, but that's because you're quite close to conscious here and therefore are more aware of the passage of time.

Another interesting fact, humans have the longest REM sleep of any animal. We spend about 25% of every night in REM sleep, while other animals only spend about 10% there. The going theory is that REM helps us deal with our social lives as well as unlinking emotional content from memories so that emotionally loaded memories stop freaking us out. This is possibly why post-traumatic stress sufferers keep revisiting the same dreams, as the mind tries to detach the emotional load from the memory time and again, but fails to do so. Those nightmares might in fact by a defense mechanism.

Sleep Isn't On Off

What is important to note here is that at no time during the night is you brain actually off. Yes, you might think it feels that way. After all, at one moment you're awake, the next moment you're not. That's what we experience and that therefore seems to be how sleep works. But it isn't.

The main reason for that – and my apologies if this gets a little abstract, but it will be worth it – is because we don't actually work with our experiences, but with our memories thereof. "Tomato, tomaaaato", you say, "What I experience is what I remember". And that seems reasonable, but that too turns out to be false. There are, as Daniel Kahneman explains in his fantastic book 'thinking fast and slow', two selves, the experiencing self and the remembering self. The thing is, we only really have access to one of them, namely our remembering self, and it isn't all that accurate.

It is possible to alter memories, implant false memories and erase perfectly good ones. In fact, every time you remember something you are not reaching back to the original memory, but the last time you remembered that memory. What do I mean with that? I mean that you take the memory out of storage, recall it and then – when you're done with it – put it back. The thing is, by doing this you risk altering it, as something in your environment might get tied up with the memory.
Similarly, while it might seem that your memories are like a movie, they are not. Instead your brain uses something called a 'peak and end' rule, where it remembers the worst or best moment and how you felt at the end to decide if something was nice or not. This can cause you to make bad choices.

For example, in one experiment participants all underwent two trails, one in which they were asked to keep their hands in unpleasantly cold water for 60 seconds, while in the other they were asked to keep their hands in the same mixture for 60 seconds and then – after some slightly warmer water was added – keep it in there for 30 seconds more. These extra 30 seconds were still unpleasant, but less so than the first 60 seconds. Now if our memories were in fact movies, the 'first' trail would be more desirable as it had the first 60 seconds and then the experiment was over, while the 'second' trail had the 60 seconds and then an additional 30 seconds of further unpleasantness.

However, when asked which experience they wanted to repeat, participants by and large chose the longer trail, as the ending of that trail was more pleasant than the other one. And that, according to the 'peak and end rule', means it was overall more pleasant. In other words, your remembering-self chose something that was actually worse for you.

And it gets worse. For around the time of sleep your memory is even less trustworthy than normal! This is because it is during sleep that our memories get written from short-term memory into long-term memory, which means around this time there is a good chance that things go wrong. For example, the last few minutes before you go (back) to sleep are actually permanently deleted from your memory.
This is something called 'retrograde amnesia' and is why you often can't remember reading that last page before you turned off the lights. It is also for this reason that you are sometimes convinced your alarm clock didn't go off when in fact it did. What happened is you woke up, turned off the alarm clock and fell back asleep, but you don't remember any of it because the memories didn't get stored properly.

Is this also why you sometimes wake up and say strange things during the night? Not exactly, though it's related (and why you won't *remember* saying them). The reason we say strange things and mumble in our sleep is because different parts of our brains switch off at different times – with some parts, like our hippocampus which is responsible for memories, going early, while others never switching off entirely. For example, our danger-monitoring mechanisms stay alert, just in case that leopard is sneaking up on us.

Our consciousness, though it doesn't feel like it, is just another (quite small) system that forms a part of our mind. You can imagine it being something like a spot light shining on that area of your mind where you should pay attention, be it work, hunger, or that itch that you just can't seem to reach. The thing is that just because your consciousness has not been turned off does not mean every part of your brain is going at full tilt. So, for example, they asked participants after they'd just woken up if they were fully awake. Even though they said yes and truly thought they were, when they were asked to do difficult logical problems they did far worse than later in the day. That part of their brain had simply not been booted up yet!

So why are you telling me this?

Not just because it's interesting (though we think it is). There are two more reasons. First of all, it means that if you're not asleep that doesn't mean you're not recuperating. Just because your conscious mind is still on doesn't mean everything else is as well. So don't stress out too much, especially as that stress will actually make it far more difficult for you to fall asleep.

And secondly, just because you remember having a bad night doesn't mean you actually had one. Your memory does crazy things and maybe you woke up at the wrong moment, thereby – according to the 'peak and end rule' – making it seem like you slept poorly, when you didn't. The reason that is important is because if you are convinced that you slept poorly, then you will feel poorly. That's what is called a self-full-filling prophecy. So when you wake up take a moment to relax, breathe deeply and take stock. Are you thinking clearly? Does your body feel rested? Perhaps if you let go of the idea that you slept badly, you'll find out that you slept much better than you did and just have bad memories (which might in fact just be dreams).

Or maybe not – maybe your memories are in fact correct. Quite often they will be. Still, it is worth a try, isn't it? After all, a moment's reflection only costs you a moment, while it might save your entire day. So give it a shot!

Chapter 2: What Causes Insomnia?

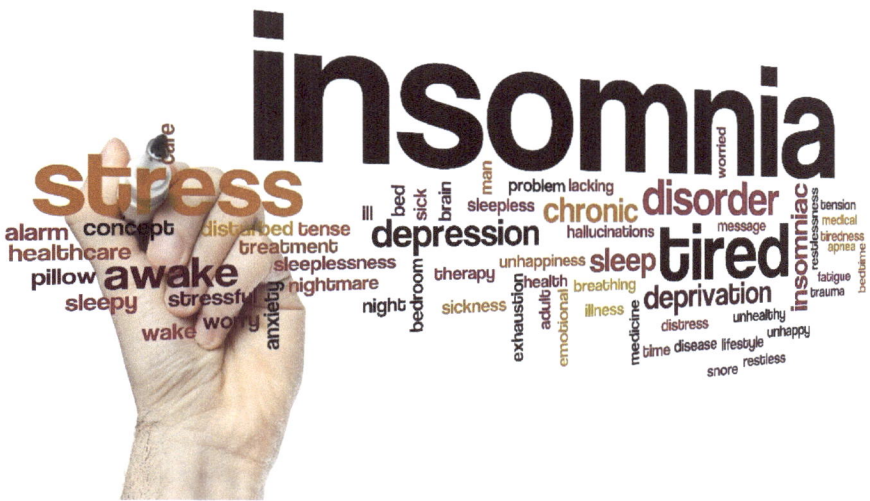

There is only so much that you can do by relativizing after the fact. Not all your bad nights are down to you remembering them as being bad. And those aren't going to go away simply through wishful thinking.

So let's explore what causes insomnia, as often knowing the cause of something can serve as the first step to eliminating it and helping you recover.

There are numerous reasons for insomnia. Here are some of the major ones. You might have a combination of causes which will all need to be tackled.

- **Stress.** Also known as the 'fight or flight' response, stress can very seriously affect your sleep if it lasts too long. There are two different kinds of stress. The temporary kind is the type that you experience just before a major event, like a test, a presentation or something else that has you worry and fret. This kind of stress happens to us all and generally isn't that harmful. Instead of focusing on reducing this stress, it is probably better to just improve your sleep hygiene and let the stress run its course. As for long-term stress, that is an entirely different kettle of fish and something that will need to be tackled. There are numerous ways to fight stress and a detailed exploration of how to reduce the effects is beyond the scope of this book. We can, however, offer a few suggestions.

  - **Mediation.** Taking some time to learn how to meditate can greatly reduce the stress you experience and thereby help you sleep better. There are numerous resources online as to how to meditate and practice mindfulness. A good place to start is here: http://marc.ucla.edu/body.cfm?id=22 as they have a list of podcasts that can help you get started on the practice.

  - **Exercise.** Exercise is a fantastic stress buster. There are numerous ways to exercise – you can go walking, do yoga or join a gym. Try out some different ways. Importantly, don't try to overdo it. Many people throw themselves off the deep end and end up hating exercise. That is counterproductive. Instead try to find something that you'll continue doing and then build it up.

- o **Friends and family.** Spending time with people you love and whose company you enjoy is a great stress buster. You don't even need to talk about the things that are stressing you out (though you can if you want to) just being in their company is often enough to release the endorphins you need to reduce the fight or flight response.

- **Anxiety.** Sometimes we just get anxious. This can be something going on in our lives, or something dispositional (as in 'that's how you're built'). A lot of people get anxious about being anxious. Can we suggest that you at least stop doing that? We know it's a hard thing to do, but you're not helping yourself by doing it. The first step to reducing the effect of the anxiety on anxiety is to accept that you might just be built that way and that your anxiety is not a sign of weakness or personal failing.

Our anxiety level largely gets set at birth, with some us having a higher setting than others. It's a bit like having blue eyes. Just accept yourself as you are and you might find that just doing that is already enough to reduce your anxiety to some extent and improve your sleep. Another strategy that seems to help is to write your anxiety away. Some people find keeping a diary and jotting down some ideas just before bed can be immensely helpful.

- **Depression.** For some people, depression leads to wanting to sleep all the time. In some way they're lucky (as lucky as you can be when you're depressed). On the other hand, there are others where being depressed can mean exactly the opposite, with them unable to nod off. This is unfortunate as the lack of sleep will probably make the depression worse. In this case the question becomes what should you tackle first, the lack of sleep or the depression? Though there is no easy answer and it is situationally dependent, the mental wellbeing that you can receive from a good night's sleep might just tip the balance in sleep's favor. This goes double as the steps towards better sleep hygiene are relatively easy to pursue. And it will give you something to focus on and hopefully succeed at – and sometimes that's all you need to start pulling your way out of that deep hole of unhappiness.

- **Medical conditions.** Chronic pain, cancer, arthritis, heart problems, lung disease and acid reflux are among illnesses that have been linked to insomnia. Unfortunately, we can't help you tackle those illnesses and though you can certainly pursue better sleep through better sleep hygiene, this will rarely tackle your underlying problems. What you really need is professional medical assistance. Still, a good night's sleep cannot be overrated so do give the sleep hygiene strategies a try.

- **Changes to your work environment or your home environment.** Some of us need stability and routine in both our work and home environments. When things change (we move offices or house, or we start sleeping with or without somebody) this can dramatically impact our sleep. In these circumstances, it will often just take time to adapt to the new situation. Rather than seeing this as a problem, try seeing it as an opportunity to change your sleeping situation and routines. After all, if change is disrupting your sleep anyway, why not use it to change your sleep situation for the better? That way, rather than forcing yourself to adapt sequentially to changes in your environment you can adapt all at once and just get it over with.

- **Lack of exercise.** We're supposed to walk, run and jump, not sit, slouch and occasionally wander to the refrigerator. For many of us not getting enough exercise can directly contribute to our sleeping problem. The best way to fight this is to start exercising. It's a straightforward enough idea that is no doubt going to inspire groans in some readers, but that doesn't make it any less true. Note that you don't immediately have to start torturing yourself for an hour in the gym. It's fine to start off slow, by walking for 20 minutes or so or going for a bike ride. Just as long as you find it slightly strenuous, it will already be beneficial. From there it's just a matter of making sure that there is a rising line in your exercise, so that you're doing a bit more every week until you're fit and healthy.

- **Medication.** Things like antidepressants, heart pills, blood pressure medication and allergy tables have all been known to impact sleep. Similarly, ADHD medication, such as Ritalin can also keep you awake at nights. Even some simple over-the-counter pain medication can have an effect as many of these contain caffeine and other stimulants. Check the package description for side-effects like insomnia (they should be listed) and try to eliminate these, provided your health isn't seriously impacted by their removal of course!

- **Alcohol, nicotine, caffeine.** Oh tell me it isn't so! Unfortunately, it is. The vast majority of vices turn out to be bad for your sleep. We'll delve into this topic in more detail under the sleep hygiene section. For now, just try to remember that this bad triad isn't going to help you sleep, especially if you have them a short time before you try to get your shut eye.

- **Eating a big meal before bed.** Mom wasn't kidding when she said having a big meal before bed could lead to nightmares and trouble sleeping. Don't take this to mean that you can't have something small to eat just before bed – a light snack can actually help some of us head off to sleep. Try something like half a turkey sandwich, a small bowl of whole-grain, low-sugar cereal, granola with milk or yogurt or a banana. It is the big meals that you want to avoid, so don't have dinner and then hit the hay.

- **Age.** It's unfortunate but true as we get older, sleep can become harder. This is particularly true if you're over the age of 60. Fortunately, it isn't completely bad news, with us also needing a little less shut eye as we age. Still, we should certainly work harder to maintain proper sleep hygiene, seeing as there isn't really that much we can do about the aging process itself. For many as they get older a routine seems to work particularly well.

- **Being a Woman.** Yes, it's true. Women are more likely to experience insomnia than men. The world simply isn't fair. As you can't really do anything about being a woman, the only real thing you can do is improve the situation under which you sleep. To make matters worse, many women experience more insomnia during pregnant and menopause. Fortunately, both of these experiences don't last forever. Unfortunately, that isn't much help when you're caught in the middle of it and haven't been able to get a good night sleep for a while. For menopause there are some hormonal treatments that can reduce the effects. You might want to consider using some of these if you're finding that it's exceptionally hard to sleep. As for pregnancy there aren't that many options, though again, practicing good sleep hygiene might help and many people find meditation useful.

- **Working shifts.** People that work strange hours are more at risk for insomnia. This problem greatly increased if their work patterns change frequently. In fact, quite a few night workers never really get used to working nights and continue to find sleeping through the day difficult. In part this is because of our biological rhythms, which we can't really change. What we can change is how much light and noise pollution we experience during the day. For that reason, invest in heavy drapes, double glazing, earplugs and other tools to reduce the effects of the day. Also try to create a standardized routine so that even though it's day time, your body is properly prepared for sleep.

- **Jet Lag.** If you travel a lot, you'll probably find that you're having trouble sleeping. Jet lag can be very frustrating, especially if you're always on the road and therefore can never really adjust to the time zone you're in. Fortunately, a lot of research is being done in how to alleviate its effects and there seems to be some suggestions that flashes of light can help alleviate the effects[2], though at this point the research only suggests the effect helps you reduce the problem if you travel west. As routines are hard to maintain on the road, try to at least get in some exercise. After all, if they're sending you all over the world, they might as well put you up in hotels with a gym!

---

[2]   https://www.theguardian.com/science/2016/feb/09/cure-for-jet-lag-a-strobe-light-in-the-eyeballs-while-you-sleep

Chapter 3: How Much Sleep Do We Need?

It is a fact that even most of the people who don't have insomnia don't sleep enough. We can put most of the blame for our sleep deprivation at the (blanket covered) feet of former misinformation. For a while, the general consensus seemed to be that you could 'practice' sleeping less and ultimately get used to it without any negative consequences. This is not true. Only 3% of the population can get by with six hours of sleep a night or less. The rest of us need more. We can't learn to get by on less and if we try to, we'll suffer the negative effects of sleep deprivation.

You should think of being awake as a budget of sorts and if you overspend this budget, you'll build up a sleep debt. If we're not careful, not sleeping enough can actually lead to brain damage, shorten our lives and negatively affect our emotional stability. This is a serious problem with the Centers for Disease Control and Prevention (CDC) saying that 35% of the population are not getting enough sleep. That's a serious number!

Don't take this to mean that you have to sleep the full hours every night and that if you occasionally can't get enough, you're dooming yourself to wasting away and mental decline. That's not the case. Not getting enough sleep one or two nights a week isn't a problem, as long as you catch up on it! Of course if you don't take the time to do that, the effects might get more severe.

This is how much sleep we actually need:
- Newborns need 16-18 hours

- Preschoolers need 11-12 hours
- School age children need at least 10 hours
- Teens need 9-10 hours
- Adults need 7-8 hours[3]
- Only 3% of the population can get by with 6 hours of sleep

Have trouble sleeping? You're far from alone. As many as 5o to 70 million people in the US alone suffer from sleep or wakefulness disorders like insomnia and sleep apnea[4]. And the fact that you've picked up this book probably means that you're one of these people. If that is the case, you might want to skip this next section, where we cover some of the basic effects of sleep deprivation. Instead jump straight to the section entitled 'sleep diary'. After all, you probably already have a pretty good idea of what not getting enough sleep does to you and you probably don't need the extra anxiety.

---

[3] http://www.cdc.gov/features/sleep/

[4] Insufficient Sleep Is a Public Health Problem
http://www.cdc.gov/features/dssleep/

Chapter 4: What Sleep Deprivation Does to You

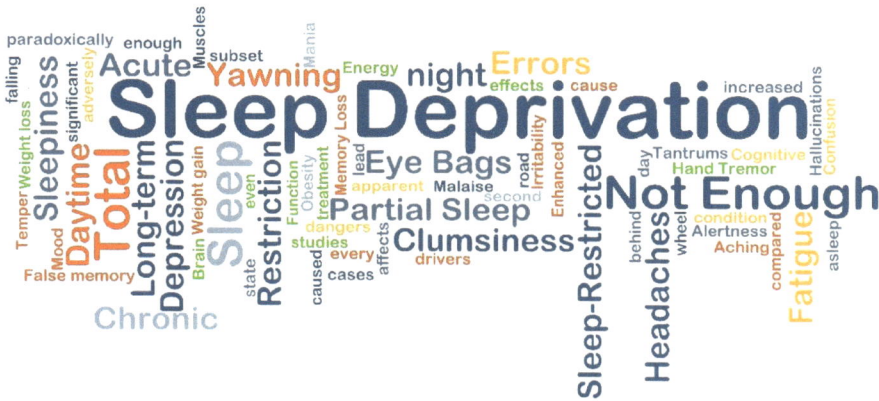

Still here? Well, there is something to be said for being well informed! Getting enough sleep has been shown to have numerous benefits, not least of which is the fact that there is nothing better for happiness – including money, friends and family, even love – than a good night's sleep. It just doesn't get much better than waking up well rested.

Furthermore, sleeping well leads to:
- Less rumination
- More emotional stability
- Better concentration
- Better health
- A better sex life
- Less pain
- Clearer thinking
- An improved immune response[5]

---

[5]   http://www.webmd.com/sleep-disorders/features/9-reasons-to-sleep-

Sleep deprivation, on the other hand can lead to:
- Reduced cognitive abilities
- Reduces muscle mass and bone growth
- Reduced self-control
- A weaker immune system
- A higher likelihood of illness
- Weight gain and overeating
- Increased risk of heart disease[6]
- Mood swings
- Memory and cognitive impairment
- Increased risk of accidents and mistakes
- Greater stress in body and mind[7]

That's quite a list, isn't it? Basically, the underlying theme here is that the body needs sleep to recuperate and reduce the negative effects of being awake – both physically and mentally. Research has even demonstrated that sleeping leads to greater skill learning with people who'd learned a task and took a nap afterwards doing better at not just memory tasks, even at motor-skill tasks. And this has nothing to do with actual sleep deprivation; this is just a side effect of sleeping after skill learning, with the brain using the sleep stage to form new mental connections and reinforce brain patterns.

In other words, you should really take the time to sleep better (and enough).

more?page=3

---

[6] http://www.healthline.com/health/sleep-deprivation/effects-on-body

[7] http://www.webmd.com/sleep-disorders/features/important-sleep-habits?page=1

Chapter 5: Sleep Diary

Don't skip over this section. It isn't exceedingly long and it is worth reading, as the sleep diary can help you figure out why you're sleeping badly and what you need to change or improve in order to sleep better.

You can choose to ignore the sleep diary and instead try applying the ideas listed in this book willy-nilly, choosing those things from the grab bag of ideas that strike you most and trying them out. There is nothing against this strategy. It might well work! The only problem is that you might well end up overdoing it, cutting out enjoyable activities that are not in fact affecting your sleep. With the sleep diary, on the other hand, you can pinpoint what it is that is actually affecting your sleep and that way only eliminate those things that you have to.

The sleep diary is a simple idea. You take five minutes in the evening to track what you did before you slept and five minutes in the morning to record how well you slept. From this you can then work out what things affect your sleep and what things really don't seem to have very much to do with it. We've even included two printable sheets to make the whole task that bit easier!

Finding it difficult to print from a eBook format? Check out this version: https://sleepfoundation.org/sleep-diary/SleepDiaryv6.pdf

How to use it

There are two sections to the diary. One labelled 'morning' the other 'evening'. They've been designed so that they're easy to use and don't take a lot of time. Obviously, they'll only really work if you fill them in! It's probably best to put them in a clear and obvious location so that you won't forget. Also, perhaps a reminder – something like a sticky note? – will help. Remember where we explained a while back how your memory isn't the same as your experience? That's important here as well. Don't wait with filling in your diary, as further removed memories are generally less accurate!

Then, when you have one or two weeks of data, you can start looking for patterns. A quick guide to a pattern – one occurrence of an activity and you sleeping poorly that night is not a pattern. We're very quick to jump to conclusions (for many people that's a favorite sport), but doing so might well end up obscuring the real problem. Wait for a problem to repeat itself several times before you determine it is a cause for your insomnia. Otherwise you might just end up blaming the wrong thing (and not actually getting any better sleep as the actual cause(s) remain at large!).

Another thing to be careful about is that you don't blame the wrong thing when activities come together. Perhaps you smoke when you drink and every time you do the combination you end up not sleeping well. In this case it could be that the smoking is making you sleep poorly. Alternatively, it could be the alcohol. A third possibility is that it's a combination.

So what to do? The easiest thing is to initially cut out one of the activities and see how that influences your sleep. If that doesn't help, then cut out the other activity as well. If you then find your sleep is improving, you could consider bringing back the original activity you cut. If you continue to sleep well, then it was the second activity that was the culprit. If you start sleeping poorly again then both activities together were to blame and you need to go back to cutting them both.

Another important point: There can be several causes for your insomnia. It could be a concert of different causes that is making you sleep badly. In other words, just because you're sleeping better doesn't mean you should end the sleeping dairy exercise. Why sleep well when you can sleep fantastically? Keep going and keep studying your sleeping patterns. The better you understand them, the more likely you'll be able to make your sleep an absolute dream!

Complete in the Morning

__/__/__	Day 1	Day 2	Day 3	Day 4	Day 5	Day 6	Day 7
Slept at: (AM/PM)							
Woke at: (AM/PM)							
Slept for __ hours:							

Last night I fell asleep (tick one per day)

Easily	☐	☐	☐	☐	☐	☐	☐
After some time	☐	☐	☐	☐	☐	☐	☐
With difficulty	☐	☐	☐	☐	☐	☐	☐

I felt (tick one per day)

Refreshed	☐	☐	☐	☐	☐	☐	☐
Somewhat refreshed	☐	☐	☐	☐	☐	☐	☐
Tired	☐	☐	☐	☐	☐	☐	☐

During the night I woke up:

# of times							
# of min. (total)							

My sleep was interrupted by:
(e.g. too hot, noise, light, allergies, people, pets, stressful thoughts)

Notes:

Complete in the Evening

_/_/_	Day 1	Day 2	Day 3	Day 4	Day 5	Day 6	Day 7

I consumed caffeinated drinks and/ or exercised for 20 minutes in the
(M)orning/ (A)fternoon/ (E)vening/ (N)one:

Caff drinks M/ A/ E/ N							
Exercised: M/ A/ E/ N							

Medication used:

Took a nap (circle one)?

Yes/ No	Y/N	Y/N	Y/N	Y/N	Y/N	Y/N	Y/N
How long?							

How likely were you to dose off during the day while doing things?
(N)o chance/ (S)light chance/ (M)oderate chance/ (H)igh chance

N/S/M/H							

My Mood today was (P)leasant/ (U)npleasant/ (H)orrible

P/ U/ H							

Two hours before bed I consumed (tick if appropriate):

Alcohol	☐	☐	☐	☐	☐	☐	☐
A heavy meal	☐	☐	☐	☐	☐	☐	☐
Caffeine	☐	☐	☐	☐	☐	☐	☐
Nicotine	☐	☐	☐	☐	☐	☐	☐

My Routine included: (e.g. read a book, used a gadget, took a bath, or listened to music)

Chapter 6: Sleep Hygiene

And now we get to the actual sleep hygiene! But wait, I hear some of you cry, "haven't you already told us what to do"? Like, reduce stress, avoid irregular work patterns and don't get jet lag? And of course you're right. Still, those were more about removing possible causes for insomnia, while here we're going to be concentrating on activities that let you sleep better overall, even if you don't have insomnia.

You see, even though you might not wake up often and getting to sleep soon after you put your head down, that does not necessarily mean you're sleeping well. Going unconscious isn't the same thing as getting the rest you need (just ask a boxer if he feels well rested after getting knocked to the mat). And so, here we're going to not just offer methods of making it easier for you to sleep and avoid waking up, but also make certain that the sleep you have is of better quality and you wake up more rested.

So how do you know if the sleep you're getting isn't good or long enough? Here's a check list of problems that might suggest that this is the case.
- You need an alarm clock to wake up on time
- You frequently use the snooze button
- Getting out of bed is a struggle
- You feel slow and sluggish in the afternoon
- You need to nap to get through the day
- You get drowsy when in meetings, lectures, warm rooms and while driving
- Similarly, heavy meals make you tired
- In the evening you fall asleep in front of the TV or while relaxing

- You feel the need to 'catch up' on sleep on the weekends
- You fall asleep almost as soon as your head hits the pillow

Are some of the above applicable to you? Well then it's time to consider changing a few things in your day-to-day (or should that be night-to-night?) life to improve the quality of your sleep.
Let's get started, shall we?

Establish a Routine

Routines don't just help you wake up in the morning. They can be just a useful habit to help you get to sleep at night. For this reason, it's important that you take some time to standardize your sleep patterns.

The first step in this process is to make certain, as much as possible, that you get to sleep at about the same time at night and wake up at about the same time as well. This will allow your body and your brain to begin the process of synchronizing your biological cycles.

Similarly, just like how reading the news in the morning might help you come more fully into the world of the wide awake, so too having certain bed-time routines will help you relax and prepare for sleepy time. What exactly these routines are will be different for everybody. Perhaps you read a book, apply a face cream, listen to classical music, tell your kids a bedtime story or stretch. It doesn't matter what it is, as long as you make sure you do it every evening so that your mental processes start recognizing it for what it is – a way to relax and go to sleep easily.

What you should not do is take actions that end up raising your excitement levels rather than lowering them. So don't do pushups, don't watch exciting television programs and don't scream at the dog or any other member of your household. Note that sex is a good exception to this rule. Yes, it gets the heart beating faster, but after it's done (provided you're satisfied, yes you can let your husband read this) you can actually end up feeling far more relaxed and this can be very beneficial for sleep.

And don't let your routines slip during the weekends! Oh no, you cry, but the weekends are for sleeping in! Well, the only reason weekends are for sleeping in is because you're not getting enough good quality sleep during the week. If you follow the suggestions in this book, that will no longer be the case. And from there you'll be able to get out of bed early yet well rested. The added bonus here is that you'll have more time on those days where that time is all yours! Not too shabby, right?

One thing to not include in your night routine is screen time, as the blueness of many devices is bad for your sleep. The reason is explained in more detail under 'get morning sun'. Suffice it to say that the blueness of the screen reminds us of morning sun[8]. So stay away from your television, your computer, your tablets and even your phones just before bed.

If that is absolutely impossible for you to do (addicted anyone?), you might want to consider buying special glasses that will filter the blueness from devises and thereby lessen the effect of screens on your night rest[9]. Some people say they make you look silly, but then who cares what you look like just before you nod off, right? And if they help, they help!

Your Bed Is for Sleeping

As the title suggests, your bed is for sleeping and you should use it exclusively for that. Keep away any situations that make you anxious, stressful or tense from where you sleep. Even events that excite you and stimulate you should be avoided as these can end up becoming associated with the place you lay down your head, thereby making it more difficult for you to wander your dreamscape.

Don't argue in your bedroom. Don't play computer games on your bed. Don't watch television either. All these things are for other parts of the house.

---

[8] http://www.webmd.com/sleep-disorders/features/power-down-better-sleep

[9]   http://well.blogs.nytimes.com/2015/04/07/can-orange-glasses-help-you-sleep-better/

The reason for this is that we are prone to connect thoughts and emotions to places and things. Seeing the fridge triggers hunger, seeing the ashtray makes us want to smoke and seeing your bed should make you want to sleep, not scream, shout or dance the tango. And the way to do that is to not do those activities near our bed. Sounds straight forward enough, right?

A good way to reduce how angry, excited and worried you get near your bed is by not bringing your phone into your bedroom with you! If you can make it a practice to only check such devices outside of your bedroom that can already make a dramatic difference to how well you sleep.

Comfort Is Vital

Some people seem to think that because they're unconscious, it doesn't matter if they're comfortable, provided they don't wake up. These people are in for a rude awakening (terrible pun, I know). How comfortable you are as you sleep most certainly changes how rested you are when you wake up. So make sure that you've got a good mattress, that your pillow is right for you and that your room temperature is neither too hot nor too cold. If you make certain you're comfortable when you're lying in bed, you'll reap the sleep dividends.

It isn't just your bed that needs to be good either. Your entire bedroom needs to be geared towards giving you the best night rest possible. So ensure that your curtains are thick enough, your room temperature is just right and that there is no noise pollution seeping in and disturbing your sleep.

If there's too much light at night in your neighborhood, there are numerous options. You can invest in heavier curtains that block out the light. If that turns out not to be enough think about investing in shutters. Do note that it is good to have light come into your bedroom in the morning as this will help wake you up (see 'get morning sun'). For this reason, it might be a good idea to set your shutters on a timer, so that they open automatically thirty minutes before you're supposed to wake up. Then the sun can act like a natural alarm clock! Much better than being alarmed, right?

An electric timer can also be useful if you prefer your bedroom to be cold while you sleep, but you don't want it to be freezing when you get up. In this case you can set the timer to kick in before you wake up. That way the room will be nice and toasty, making it a bit easier (and nicer) to climb out of bed.

Double glazing is another thing to consider for your bedroom (and the rest of your house) as it can both keep your room warmer and serve to keep out unwanted sound. If sound is a big problem in your neighborhood, consider earplugs. A lot of people really don't like the idea until they try them. Modern day earplugs are so comfortable you really barely feel them (this is not a lie – a friend of ours has worn them into work on more than one occasion because he simply forgot they were there). For the light sleeper who's easily bothered by noise, they can be a godsend.

What You Drink and How You Sleep

Not just caffeine but also alcohol affects your night rest. You probably knew about caffeine. It is a stimulant and thereby makes it harder for you to drift off. What you might not have known is that this can be true for up to four hours after you've had your last cup. Yes, that means that even a cup you had before dinner can negatively influence your night rest. So don't be tempted to have any coffee, soft drinks, tea or (god forbid) energy drinks in the evening! They might taste good but is that really worth tossing and turning and watching the minutes tick by?

Similarly, for those who have trouble sleeping, alcohol is a no go – and that's not just because you might end up with hungover! You see, though it does knock you out initially, which can make it seem a worthwhile tool to get you to sleep, it adversely affects your sleep. This is in large parts down to two reasons. The first is that alcohol upsets your internal thermostat. It thereby leads to your body going through hot and cold spells, which will lead to you tossing and turning as you first throw off the blankets and afterwards go scrambling around to get them back again.

Secondly, it negatively impacts your REM sleep[10]. As mentioned earlier, this is an important stage of your sleep where a great deal of mental processing happens that you need this in order to feel refreshed. It is also vital for laying down memories and skill learning. Finally, it also increases the risk of sleep walking, sleep talking and snoring.

---

[10] http://www.webmd.com/sleep-disorders/news/20130118/alcohol-sleep

Need more reasons not to drink in order to sleep? Well, you can become dependent and in that situation you're stuck in a vicious circle where you can't sleep without alcohol but it makes you sleep worse, thereby aggravating the problem.

Note that the not drinking thing doesn't just stop with alcohol and caffeine. Also be aware that other liquids can disturb your night rest by making your sleep less comfortable (you know that full bladder feeling) and making it more likely you'll have to get up during the night. This doesn't mean you should allow yourself to get dehydrated, but it's better to have a few sips of water rather than knock back several glasses. Keep that for the morning, when a trip to the bathroom isn't as much of a problem.

Get Up to Get to Sleep

The standard wisdom seems to be that if you want to get to sleep, you have to stay in bed and keep trying, even if you're not having any luck. This might not actually be such a good idea. The thing is, the longer you are in bed unable to get to sleep, the harder it can become to get to sleep. In part, this is because you'll end up becoming more and more frustrated with your inability to sleep. Also, your body might just not be ready for sleep yet. So get up, let your sleep attempt reset and try again 20 minutes later, as on average that will mean you'll be able to get to sleep sooner.

What to do in those 20 minutes? Well, don't turn on the television, don't check your email and don't grab your phone to play the newest trending game. Stay away from screens and anything that is exciting. Instead, try a book, a moment relaxing in a comfortable chair or a short walk, provided the night isn't too cold and the streets aren't too busy. It doesn't have to be too long. Just enough to reset yourself, so that when you return to bed you can start over without your first failed attempt haunting you.

Exercise Is Exhausting

You probably knew about this one even before we mentioned it earlier in the book, but it is worth mentioning again. Exercise is a fantastic way to improve your night rest and should definitely be on your list of activities to undertake if you're not sleeping well – to not even talk about the other health benefits!

Want numbers? Alright, they conducted research at the Northwestern University's Department of Neurobiology and Physiology into this phenomenon and found that just doing aerobic exercises four times a week for at least 20 minutes had people who slept poorly state that their sleep went from 'poor' to 'good'[11].

---

[11]   http://www.northwestern.edu/newscenter/stories/2010/09/aerobic-exercise-relieves-insomnia.html

They didn't need to do anything else! That sounds pretty convincing, right? The only thing you've got to watch out for is that you don't exercise in the two hours before bed. Then it once against becomes counterproductive (there is always a catch isn't there?).

Get Morning Sun

We have these things called 'circadian rhythms'. Really that's just a fancy way of saying that we have natural cycles that we go through every day for waking and sleeping. These rhythms are largely determined by the different coloration of sunlight, as these were a good short hand for our brains to know what time it was. (Electric light is evolutionarily novel and we haven't yet managed to adapt to it).

How does this work? It turns out that the morning sun and the evening sun are different in coloration due to the earth's spin and the way that short and long wavelengths refract differently when they enter the atmosphere. Okay, that sounds complicated, but it doesn't actually matter so much – what matters is that bluer light tells our brain to wake up and light towards the red end of the scale tells us to go to sleep.

And that means that if we can get sun in the morning, we can reset our rhythms and thereby make certain that we wake up when we're supposed to and start feeling tired at the time we need to. It doesn't just end there either, as the advantages of sunlight are legion. For example, it will help improve your mood and sense of wellbeing. In other words, it's better than coffee! And we're not just saying that. It is actually true. In addition, you don't have to cut out coffee in order to have more sun and you're golden. So when you wake up and you've brewed your perfect cup of black heaven, drink it by a window! It doesn't matter if it's overcast, you're still getting sunlight (though admittedly less).

Oh yes, and don't wear sunglasses during this time. The sun receptors (i.e. the things that measure the blueness and the redness of the light) are in your eyes and so sunglasses interfere with the synching of your natural rhythms. And no, you don't need your sunglasses. We got by perfectly well without them for 99.9% of our evolutionary history, so you can get by without them now!

Chapter 7: Sleep Apnea and Snoring

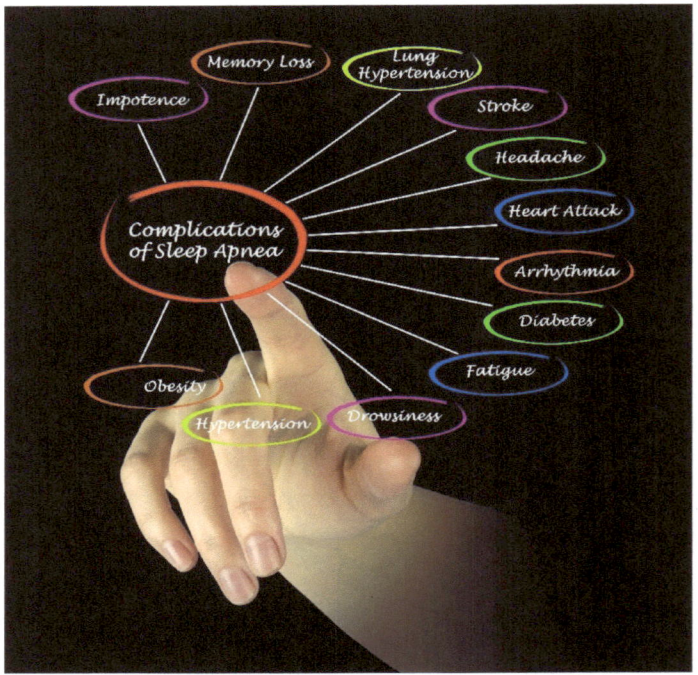

Okay, it isn't insomnia, but it can nonetheless impact your sleep almost as much. And that means that even if you've beaten the insomnia dragon, you might still not be able to get a good night's sleep. So we're quickly going to say a little bit about sleep apnea and snoring.

What is sleep apnea? It is where you momentarily stop breathing or have trouble breathing. Snoring, or what we like to call 'moonlighting as a lumberjack' is a common example of sleep apnea, though it is not the only one.

One form of sleep apnea is called 'central sleep apnea' and it is where you simply stop breathing. The second form is where your breathing passageways become blocked. This form is known as obstructive sleep apnea. Both can lead to you not getting enough air, which can make it feel like you're suffocating. That's deeply uncomfortable whether you wake up at night or not.

Central sleep apnea, which accounts for about 20% of sleep apnea cases, happens when your lungs and your brains don't communicate properly. There can be many reasons for this, including medication, strokes, surgery, Parkinson's disease and heart attacks. If you regularly take codeine, morphine or oxycodone you might experience it.

If you think there is a chance you or a loved one has this, you should really speak to a healthcare professional as it can be indicative of other health problems which can become much more severe if they are not tackled. Read more about it at the Healthline[12].

Obstructive sleep apnea, in the meantime, can happen either because your air passages are constricted or because loose skin temporarily blocks your airways. Commonly it leads to snoring, though sometimes people might not breathe for a while and then suddenly gasp for breath. Both can be very disconcerting to hear, to not even mention how bad they feel for the sufferer! After all, the brain will interpret this shortness of breath as some kind of problem, thereby negatively affecting sleep even if you don't wake up. It isn't just a brain problem either, as snoring is like carrying around a five-pound weight on your chest the entire night.

---

[12] http://www.healthline.com/health/sleep/central-sleep-apnea#Overview1

And that while it isn't that hard to do something about snoring! For example, if you're overweight, weight loss can lead to significant improvements, with 70% of snorers stopping when they shed the weight! It can also be related to sleeping on your back. Try putting a pillow under the hollow of your back to prevent yourself from turning and you might already find yourself snoring less.

Two more things that can contribute to snoring are smoking and drinking. Drinking causes the muscles in your airways to relax, which makes it more likely that skin will hang down and obstruct your breathing. Smoking, in the meantime, causes inflammation and that means there is less space for the air to get through. Oh those poor vices. They really can't get ahead anymore nowadays.

Want to know more about snoring? Check out Healthline.com[13] and WebMD[14] or contact your healthcare professional. It really is worth it!

---

[13] http://www.healthline.com/health/healthy-sleep/effective-snoring-remedies#2

[14] http://www.webmd.com/sleep-disorders/guide/snoring

Conclusion

So what is the take home message here? In a nutshell it is, if you're sleeping badly you can do something about it. There are many things that can negatively affect your sleep that you can remove and there are quite a few ways to positively impact it as well. All you need to do is take action. And that action does not need to be grabbing for the pill bottle. Pills are an option, but they should only be one of last resort. After all, as most of these medicines haven't been on the market that long, it is hard to know what the long term effects of them are. More importantly, the pill road is often a one-way street. Once you go down it, it is hard to go back as you may develop a dependency.

A much better idea is to improve your health through such activities as getting enough exercise and taking the time to reduce both your stress and anxiety. The great thing about many of the activities listed here is that they don't just benefit your sleep, they'll benefit you in many other ways as well. In this way every aspect of your life will improve. That doesn't sound too bad, right?

Finally, there is a lot to be said for attitude. Don't see yourself as a victim. Victims are at the end of a string of events and don't have any control over the situation. Instead try to see yourself as a protagonist, somebody who has control over their situation and can do something about changing what is bad in their lives.

The idea of control is important. In a famous study, psychologists exposed two groups of participants to an annoying noise that they didn't want to hear. One group had no control. They simply had to bear it. The other group was told that they could hit a button at any time to turn off the noise, but to please not do so as then the experiment would be rendered null and void. How many people in the second group actually hit the button? Zero. And yet they experienced far less stress that the first group. In other words, just the idea that they had control – even though they didn't use it – was enough to make the situation more bearable.

It is all down to mindset. Believe you can overcome your insomnia and you probably will. Believe it has the upper hand and it probably does. So be the hero in your own insomnia story and you're one step closer to beating the insomnia demons.

Good luck and good night!

How to Fall Asleep – Infographic

How To Fall Asleep

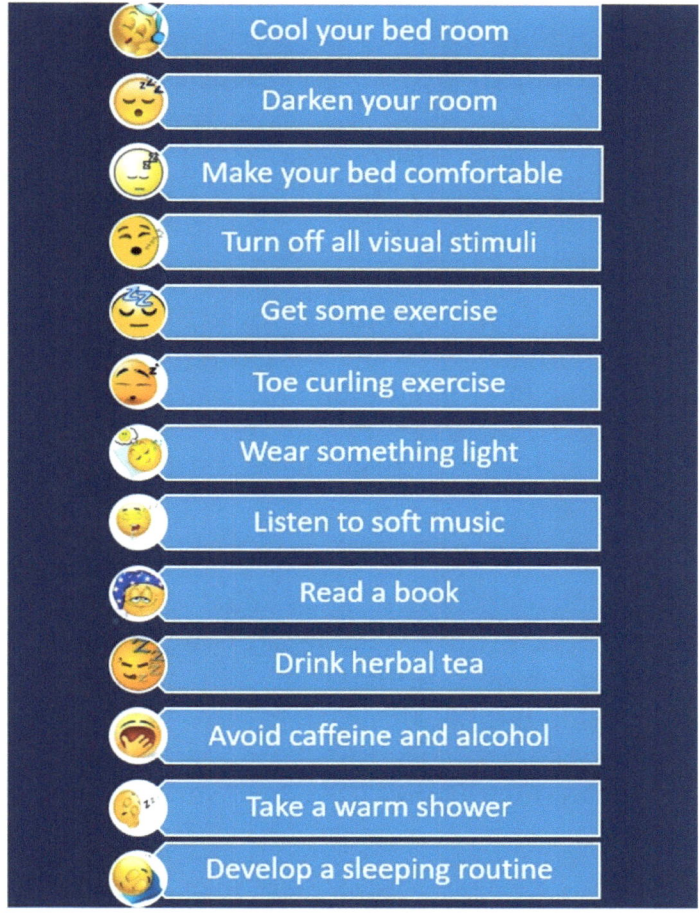

- Cool your bed room
- Darken your room
- Make your bed comfortable
- Turn off all visual stimuli
- Get some exercise
- Toe curling exercise
- Wear something light
- Listen to soft music
- Read a book
- Drink herbal tea
- Avoid caffeine and alcohol
- Take a warm shower
- Develop a sleeping routine

Check Out Other Books

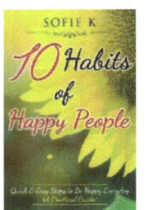	10 Habits of Happy People: Quick & Easy Steps to Be Happy Everyday (A Practical Guide) ASIN: B01CM7951S http://goo.gl/1RRKYM ISBN-13: 978-1530431939
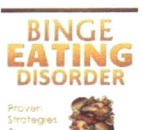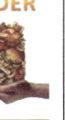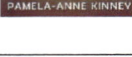	Binge Eating Disorder: Proven Strategies & Treatments to Stop Over Eating ASIN: B011QYCCNG http://goo.gl/EahwVs ISBN-13: 978-1519547088
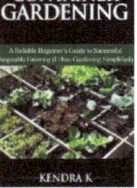	Container Gardening: A Reliable Beginner's Guide to Successful Vegetable Growing (Urban Gardening Simplified) ASIN: B014AO0JMK http://goo.gl/2C0nIw ISBN-13: 978-1517773762
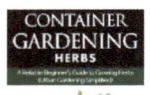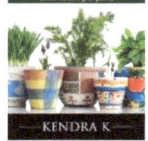	Container Gardening: A Reliable Beginner's Guide to Growing Herbs (Urban Gardening Simplified) ASIN: B015G6ZVO2 http://goo.gl/Uaoh4t ISBN-13: 978-1517646363

www.ingramcontent.com/pod-product-compliance
Lightning Source LLC
Chambersburg PA
CBHW040326010626

45792CB00024B/2172